Journey to Self & Healing

ADREANNA BARRIOS

Journey to Self & Healing by Adreanna Barrios

Copyright © 2020 Adreanna Barrios

All rights reserved. No portion of this book may be reproduced in any form without written permission from the publisher or author, except as permitted by U.S. copyright law. The moral rights of the author have been asserted.

Written in Newark, New Jersey

www.adreannabarrios.com

Ebook ISBN: 978-1-7352266-1-3
Paperback ISBN: 978-1-7352266-0-6

Library of Congress Control Number:
2020909130

Cover and illustrations by Adreanna Barrios
Photo reference by ©iStock.com/KateLeigh, (page 30)
Photo reference by ©iStock.com/PeopleImages, (page 43)

This book holds suggestions that the author has chosen to follow and share in the form of a guide. The author is not a healthcare provider. The author is providing this book and its contents on an "as is" basis and makes no warranties of any kind with respect to this book or its contents. This book is not intended as a substitute for the medical advice of physicians. The reader should regularly consult a physician in matters relating to his/her health and particularly with respect to any symptoms that may require diagnosis or medical attention.

This book was intended as a

guide to assist in self-repair.

It is a combination of

a journey once-lived

meeting up with

the person you are now.

Take a step forward.

This path may lead you

to where you need to be.

The Journey

The Very Beginning
    Sometimes to move forward...   3
    The struggle makes you, you.   4
    Breathe in. Breathe out.   7
    Believe   8

Baby Steps
    You will fall. Get Back Up.   12
    We've Been Here Before   14
    Okay. This is going to get messy.   16
    Release   18

Tough Love
    Strength and Vulnerability   22
    Okay, Let's Talk.   24

Feeding Your Soul
    Mantra   28
    Boundaries   29
    Light   30

Unwind
    Forgive   34
    Forgive Yourself   36
    Take A Break   39

Moving Forward
    Be Humble   42
    Accept   44
    Be Open   46

Remember Me?
    Triggers   50
    Unspoken   52
    Self Sabotage   55

The "L" Word
    Love Yourself   58
    Accepting Love   60
    Let it Go   62
    A Home Within Yourself   64

If You Get a Little Lost
    Remember   69

A Message
    Message from the Writer   75

Glossary
    Glossary   79

The Very Beginning

Sometimes to move forward you have
to take a couple of steps back.

Let's start from the beginning. This may take a little bit of work but let's find your inner child.

Focus in and
remember the parts of you
that began *you*.

Even if the memories have been blocked
let's find them together and remember.

Were you a strong firecracker
or shy and silent
or somehow both?

At what point was there a shift in this young life's innocence? Were you once brutally silenced or forced to speak loudly outside of your comfort zone?

Think about these young memories and keep the feeling and image of the child you picture in your head. When you are ready, we can move *forward*.

The struggle makes you, **you**.

It's not easy to think about the vulnerable state of our younger selves. This feeling of bareness and vulnerability can linger with us, even as adults.

Hiding it only keeps it buried within us and our subconscious, at all times.

Why don't we deal with it?

While remembering your young, more innocent self, you may notice a need to save that person from trouble or heartbreak. Any moment, big or small, could've greatly impacted that child's way of dealing with the world and his or her emotions. Maybe that child needed someone to help them recover from an unfortunate event.

Here's your chance to save that person
and that part of yourself.

Remember the face that held all of your innocence and pureness and remember what took it away. Now find a safe place for your inner child. Tell him or her of how precious they are. Remind that young, scared face of how **worthy** they are.

Say it out loud.

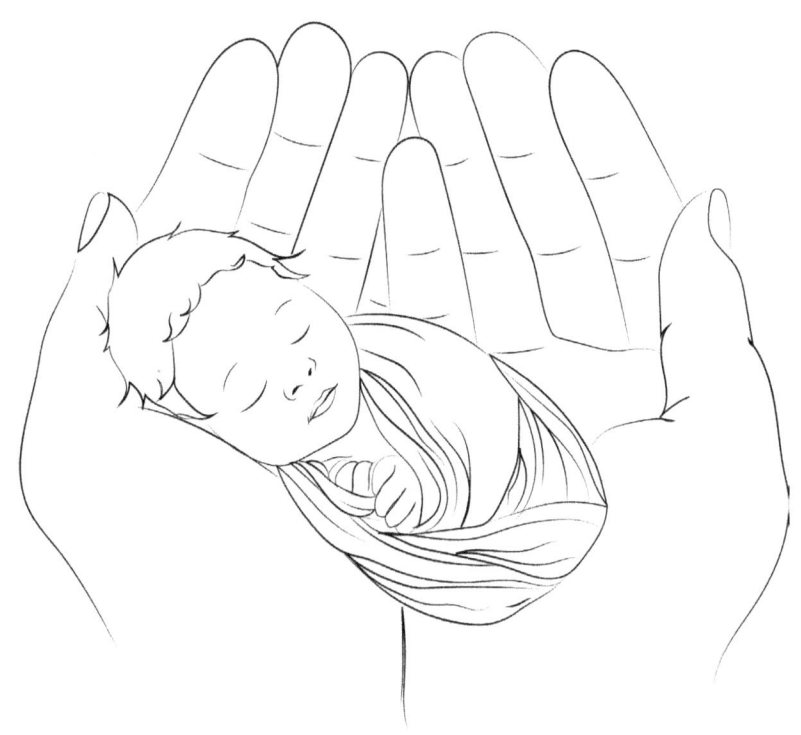

You're safe.

Remind the child of what they did not realize then but of what you are aware of now.

You're strong.

Now, hold on to that feeling.

Breathe in. Breathe out.

You have done a lot of work looking into your past. You may feel a little relieved but also a little nervous. This is perfectly fine.

A part of you and your past that you've been holding on to for so long has finally evolved. A part of you has gotten so much stronger.

Today, you can relax.

Allow your mind and body time to readjust to the person you know you are now. Allow yourself a chance to go through the rest of the day with just a little less weight on your shoulders. Even if you wish to revisit the past or future - attempt to do so in a calm way.

Allow yourself to
accept your **strength** and how far you've come as a person.

You've grown a lot.
You've been through enough.

Now, we can put those negative thoughts to rest.

Believe

Connect with your spiritual self.

Practice things that make you feel happy, humble, and whole.

If you follow a religious belief - it may be time to embrace some practices that bring you to a place where your soul and mind connect.

If not - you can still practice things that will help bring your self a sense of

                    peace.

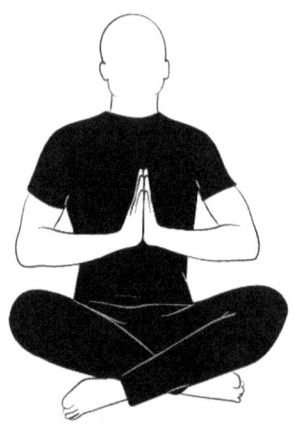

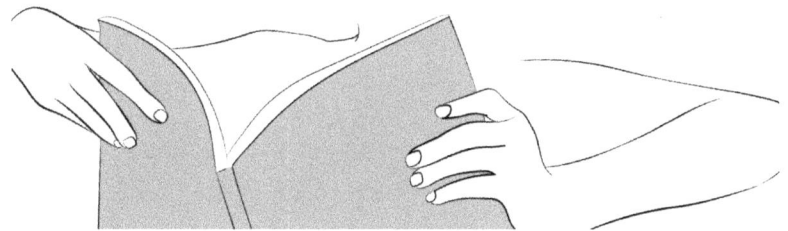

Some things that help the mind and soul are painting, drawing, playing an instrument, meditating, singing, gardening, and talking to a loved one - even catching up on that show you used to love.

Things that can help the body, mind, and soul are things that involve moving (yes, exercise) such as yoga, walking, dancing, and swimming.

While I want to connect with you emotionally and mentally, things like this can also help you feel more connected with yourself. They can remind you of your purpose and help to guide you on your journey. Most importantly, things like this will remind you of your

                strength.

Baby Steps

You will fall. Get Back Up.

The path to healing isn't a straight line.
There are times when you may even feel like you are going backwards and this is part of the process, believe it or not.

Healing takes time.
There will be good days.
There will be bad days.

Let's prepare.
Remember:

Even toddlers fall hundreds of times
And continue to get back up

                                                      And get back up.

Until one day,
They are finally

                                                      Standing up.

Until one day,
They learn something new.

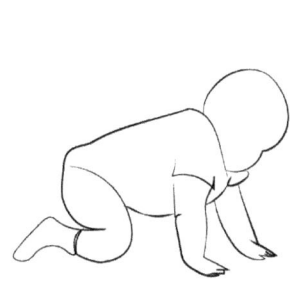
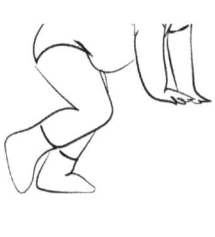

                  And they're walking.
              Then, they're running.

And you. You're going to fall.
You've fallen before.
But just like before -

                          Get Back Up.

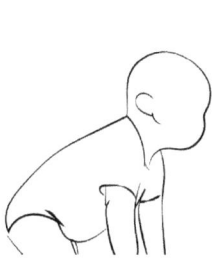
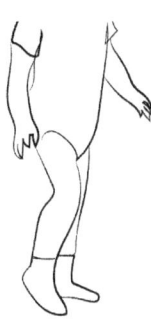

We've Been Here Before

Allow me to address something
you may have missed.

You

have stumbled before.

You

have been in a place where you
knew *nothing* before.

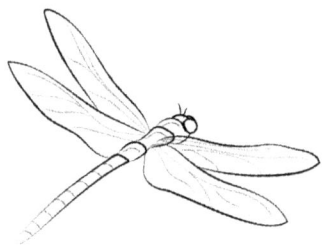

I'm not being hard on you
        or, maybe I am...

      ...but   you   will   ***soar.***

Okay. This is going to get messy.

So there's been a lot of change in your routine lately
and you still feel a little bothered.

There's still some weight on your shoulders
and some heaviness in your chest.

You know what it is.

>You need to get it off your chest.

>Confront the situation.

>Reach out to the person
>you pushed away from
>but can't escape pain from.

>Let out what you've been holding in
>for so long
>for someone else's benefit.

Release yourself from the burdens you hold on to.

Stop believing that all this weight is something

with your name on it

that you're supposed to hold *in* and take care of.

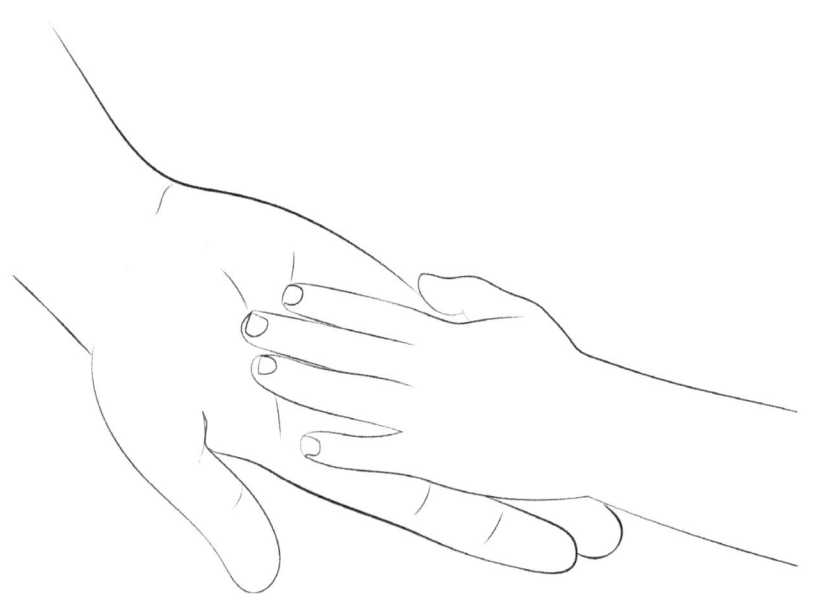

You are entitled to some peace.

You're more so able to forgive now. You can let go of so much that you've held on to for so long.

You can also repair:

>your relationships,

>yourself,

>your mind.

Release

You've put the blame on someone else and have allowed yourself to release the demons caged inside of you. It seemed you had everything under control for a while but, let's be honest,

everything you held inside...

maybe out of fear of letting go,
maybe for everyone else's protection,
maybe even out of pride

...was just creating more monsters inside of you.

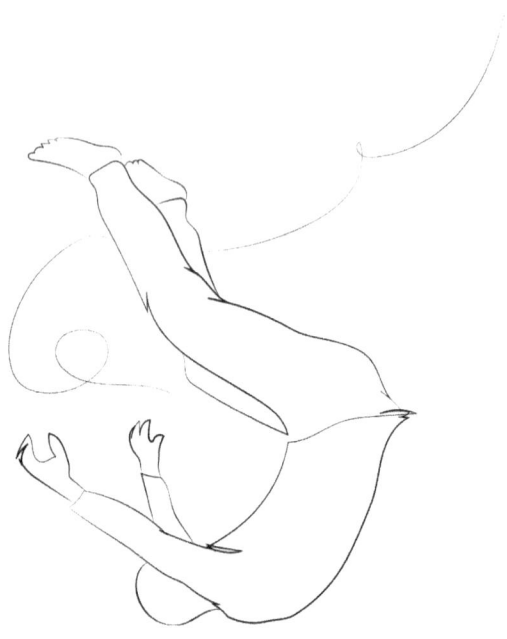

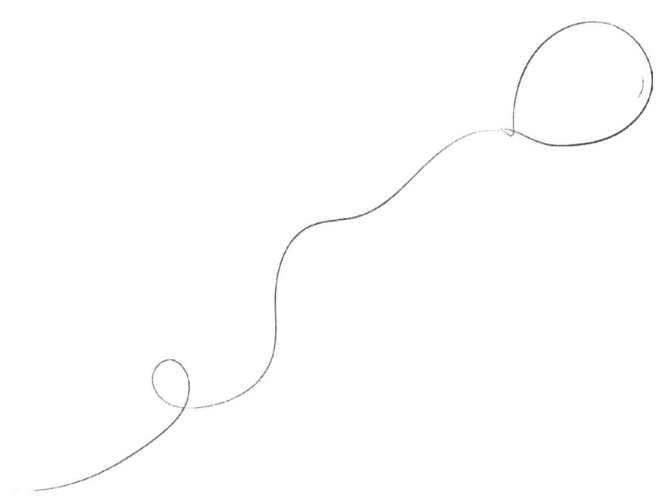

Releasing this may have resulted in an ugly and uncomfortable state of being but

> it had to be done.
>
> More importantly,
>
> you needed to be heard.
>
> *Even if you felt everything was misunderstood*
>
> you stood up for yourself
>
> and that burden
>
> is no longer yours.

Tough Love

Strength and Vulnerability

For someone who has bottled so much in for so long, it can feel frustrating to let things out. You can feel pretty *small* when sharing your *feelings* with someone out loud.

Showing actual emotion, like anger or sadness, and being heard or watched as you present your **bare** feelings can be hard.

At one point,
holding all of this in is what may have led you to believe
that's what made you strong.

It did make you strong
but it also added so much baggage.

Do you feel *lighter* now?

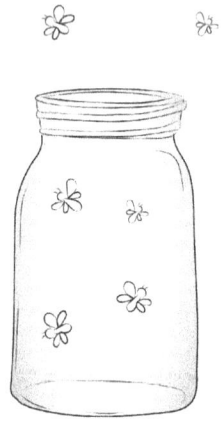

It's okay to be vulnerable.

At this point,
why not try

to be strong without so much *weight*?

You may find that it'll be easier
to think clearer and move faster with less baggage.

Okay, Let's Talk.

So you've confronted the heartless and self-centered.

And that was **a lot**.

But have you confronted yourself?

Let's face it.
You haven't been the best to yourself.

If we're going to play the blame game we have to make sure we take a good look at ourselves and the role we've played in our **toxicity**.

No more
bottling things up inside.

No more
saying *I'm not good enough.*

No more
saying *I deserve this*
when you know it's no good for you.

No more
destroying yourself
for someone else's benefit.

No more.

You said it to someone else,
now say it to yourself:

        Enough is enough.
        You deserve better.

Feeding Your Soul

Mantra

We've taken so much out of you - now what?
What will you hold on to? What is left of you?

Who are you?

You are beautiful.

You are everything.

You are **more** than

- more than -
your past, darkness, worries, or angst.

You are capable

- capable of -
*understanding, smiling, living, loving,
breathing, feeling, forgiving,
giving, and accepting.*

You are worthy.

You are light.

Boundaries

The word in itself can be pretty intimidating, I know.

What are boundaries?

Well, let's make this as breezy as possible.

Anything that will make all of this hard work
seem insignificant
should be re-examined.
(Read that again.)

Anything - or anyone -
getting in the way of your peace
should be stopped.

*Include yourself
and old ways of doing things.*

Protect yourself.
Don't over-think it.

*If it was good enough for the old you,
 if it doesn't sit right with you now,
  if it makes you feel small, or without value,*

it must be stopped.

Show yourself what you're made of.

Light

It's funny thinking back to the beginning…
Yes, I know we started at the beginning - in the beginning -

but

it feels *different* somehow now, doesn't it?

There was once this light in you that shined so bright.
You may have been too innocent to notice
the flame and sparks held - not only inside of you -
but so easily transmitted to others.

You may have forgotten...

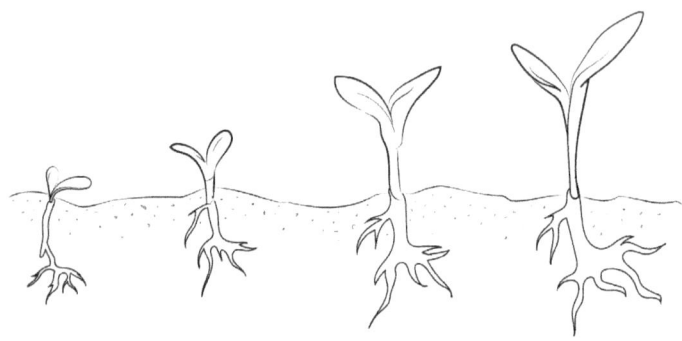

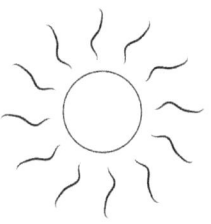

        You are light.

A lot of walls have been torn
down and it's easier to
see now.
        You are light.

A lot of weight and pain
has been passed on
and your feet don't drag as much.

        You hold light.

A lot of darkness has been
removed and filled with the
warmth inside of you.

        You are a flame.

Your look, your vibe,
your touch can be felt
by anyone now.

        You were always *light*.

Unwind

Forgive

Forgiving can be hard.

Anger is something we like to hold on to. It makes us feel *stronger* somehow.

The truth is: holding on to that grudge is only hurting you more.

It's time to forgive

for yourself.

It might sound strange but

you **deserve**
to forgive
the person that hurt you.

You deserve to feel

less weight on your shoulders.

It's just a suggestion
and, for now, it can just be a thought.

Forgive Yourself

Now, you can forgive yourself.

You can forgive yourself for any guilt you've held inside,

> *for things you've said to others,*
> > *for anything you've done*
> > > *out of pain or anger or even out of spite.*

It is your time to heal

and **let go**.

You don't need to hurt yourself anymore.

No more thinking back
and saying,

> *I should have done this.*
> *I could have done that.*

No more.

You are forgiven.

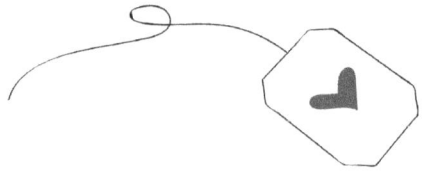

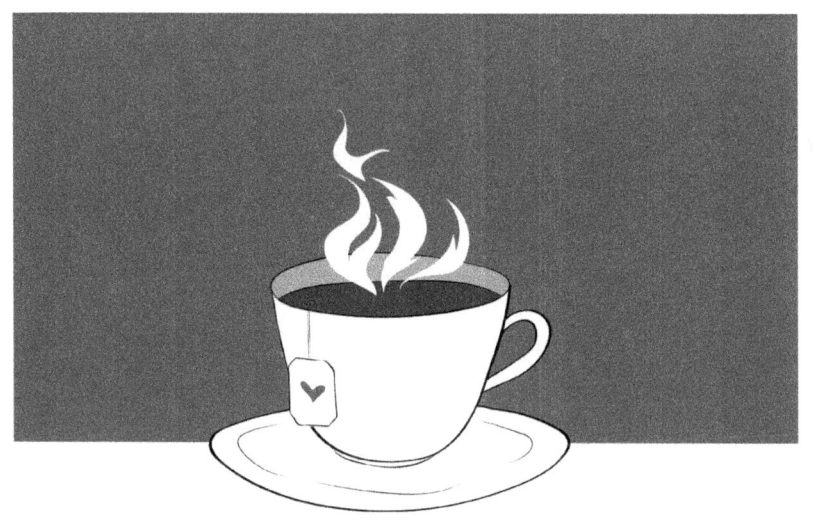

Forgiveness can be hard.
This may not be a one-step process.

Just thinking about the idea of it (over and over again)
may be what will lead you there when you least expect it.

Don't be so hard on yourself.

u n w i n d

Take A Break

Don't forget to take a break from time to time.

Healing takes a lot out of us.
For days, we can feel great, while other times we can fall into a weird *space* again.

Sometimes we just need to take a break

from thinking about it all

and recharge.

Just because you stop thinking about the *usual* things does not mean that you are no longer healing.

Feeling uncomfortable with yourself at this time does not mean that anything is wrong with you.

This is actually a **good** thing.

You can become so accustomed to the feeling of being weighed down that anything else may just feel wrong; but do not forget

the goal was to feel

different,

to feel better.

Moving Forward

Be Humble

Be thankful.

You have overcome so much on this journey.

If someone needs your help - and it doesn't cross your new boundaries - consider offering a hand or ear or even a part of your story.

*(This does **not** mean at your expense.
This still means within what feels safe to you.)*

When you feel better,
don't look at others who haven't quite made it to where you are yet as *less than* yourself.

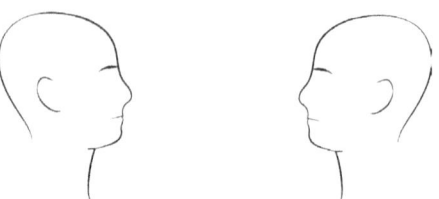

Don't get angry at an older version of yourself.

Remember there was a time when **you** were at your worst and that moment brought you to the person you are now.

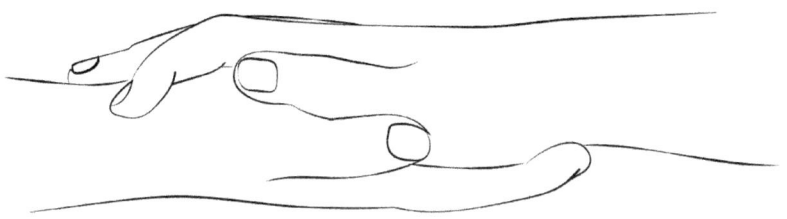

Stay humble and continue on your journey to find yourself.
Be kind to others who show signs of deep pain.

Accept

By now, a part of you
may have come to terms with

accepting the past.

The times that were hard on you
can now be viewed as stepping stones
that got you here

to who you are now.

With this in mind, you can
be proud of yourself.

You made it this far.

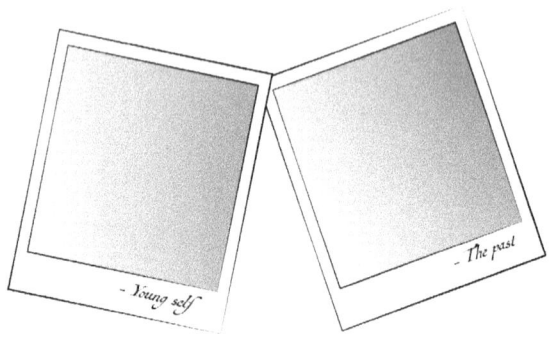

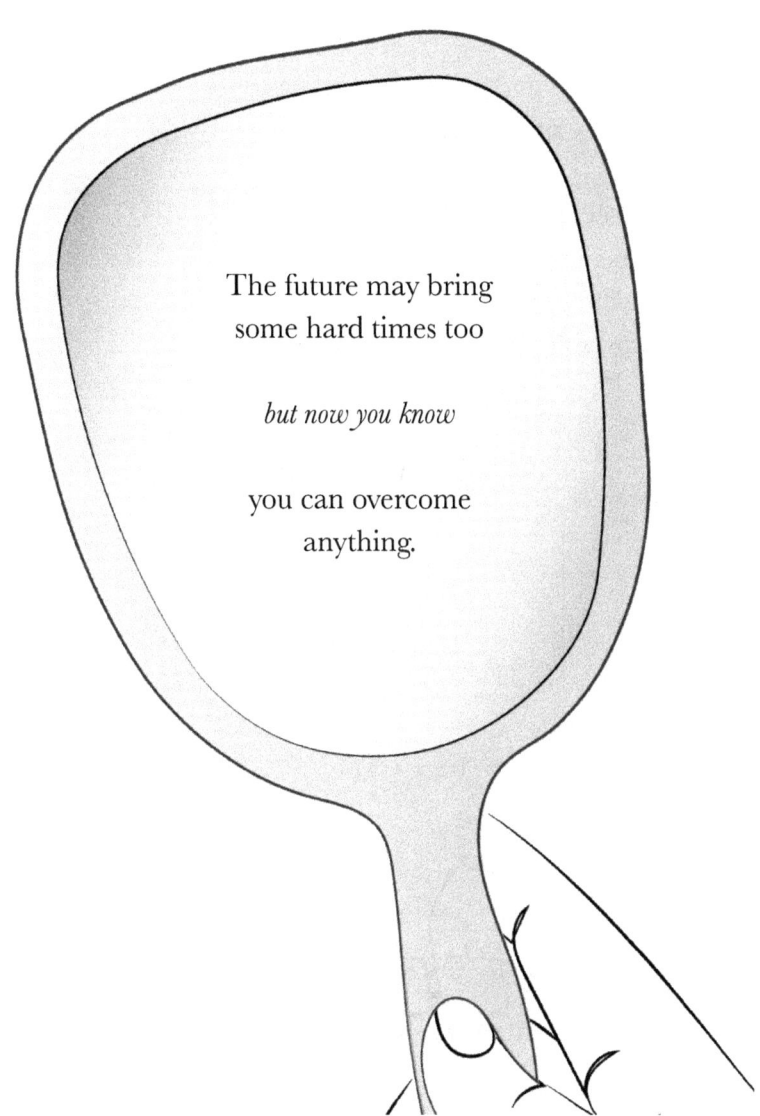

The future may bring
some hard times too

but now you know

you can overcome
anything.

Be Open

Be open
      to new people.

Be open
      to new situations.

As previously mentioned,
new may feel uncomfortable
but what you were once used to
and comfortable with - is **not** what is okay.

                You will be okay.

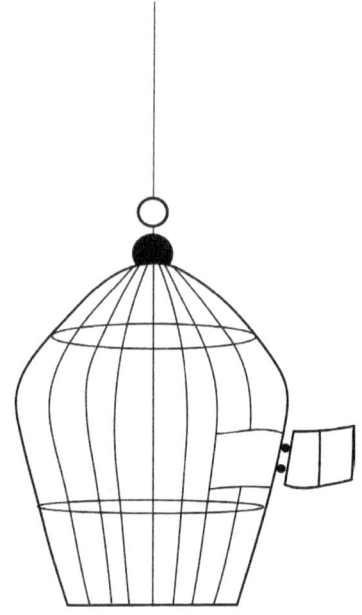

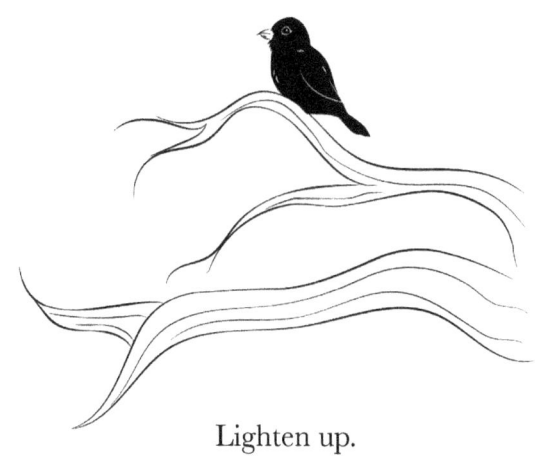

Lighten up.

(It's alright to be scared.)

Get out of your comfort zone.

Experience everything you've ever wanted.

There's a **new** world of possibilities waiting for you.

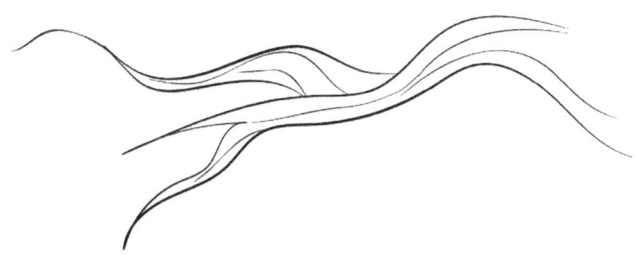

Remember Me?

Triggers

Triggers can take you *back* into
a moment and place that feel exactly
like you got thrown right into the past.

They can instantly
take over and change your mood.
They can change the way your
setting feels and looks.

A person may even
feel like *someone else*
to you - like someone who
hurt you before - like a **bad** guy.

These moments are not for the weak.
But wait...

You are **not** weak.

You are not in *that* place.

This is not that situation.

Take a second to evaluate.

*What - or who -
triggered you?
And why?*

Is this situation good for you?

Is this person good for you?

*Or are you acting
out of fear?*

Finding a way
to calm down and clear your mind
is what is best in these situations.

*This is something that is easier said than done
but believe in yourself.
You can do this.*

You can figure out what caused you to panic and *why*,
and learn how to slowly avoid
and **control** your triggers.

You can get through this.

These triggers are the strings that tie your past, present self, and future.

Unspoken

There are moments
that may have you wondering
about a conversation that you wanted
with someone that is - or seems - unreachable.

A similar feeling could be had for a conversation that
never seems to go according to plan - ending with
you feeling misunderstood.

>*In these moments,*
>*do not give up hope.*

There may be things that you still need to process
or get **off** your chest.

>There are ways to let it out.

Reach out now
to who's available to you.

This could be a family member or friend.
This could be a counselor.
This could be someone in one of your supportive circles (or
even, if you follow a religion, a member of your group).

If these suggestions don't quite feel like an appropriate outlet, then you can try to write your feelings out and:

read them out loud,

read them to a friend,

(if you are ready)

*read, text or even email them
to the person you've wanted to confront,*

*or read them, then rip and throw
that paper away when you feel comfortable
enough to let go of those emotions.*

Whatever you do, allow yourself the peace of mind to release those feelings and keep **moving** forward.

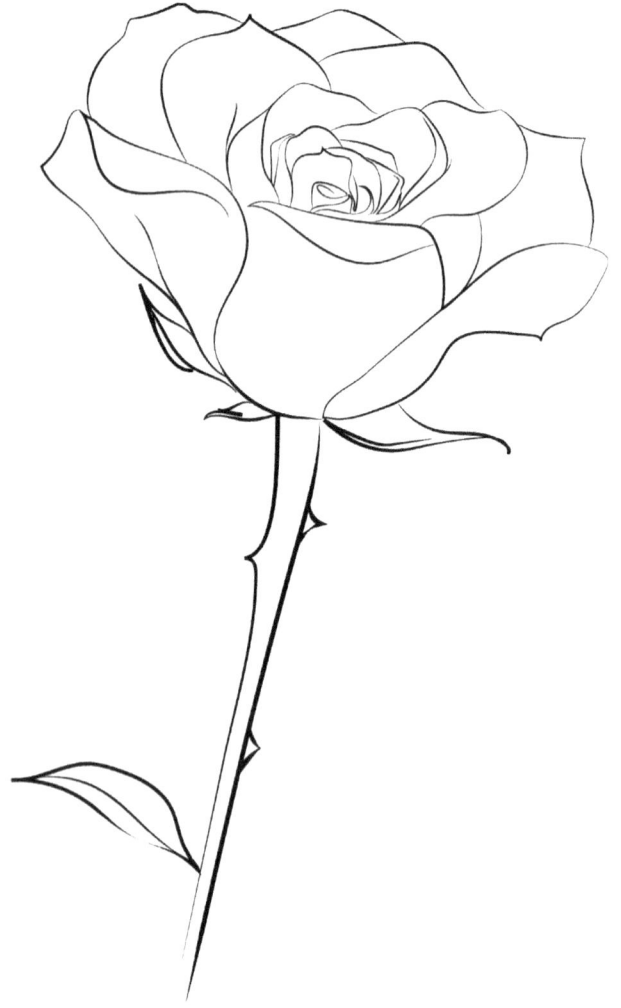

Self Sabotage

To dig deeper into the unfamiliar,
let us further address the discomfort that you may feel
with your growing self.

When things seem to actually be going okay for you in life,
it is possible to suddenly find yourself in disbelief
and in a paranoid state of **mind**.

The thought that you don't deserve happiness may
secretly linger inside.

It only makes sense to be skeptical of the new
grounds you have found yourself in but

these are your grounds.

You made this happen.

After so much progress, do not push yourself
back into a hole.

Take a breath.

You got this.

You are worth so much more.

The "L" Word

Love Yourself

You've made it this far.
I believe that you can handle the word

love.

The love you give yourself
is also the love you teach others to give you.

Be kind to yourself.

Be patient with yourself.

You - survivor of trauma - are capable of loving and that

includes **yourself**.

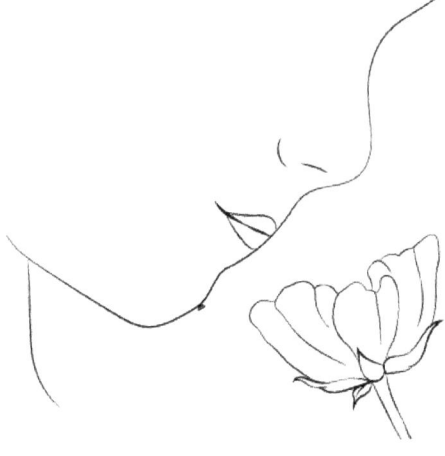

What is there to love?

Your beauty
Your strength
Your will
Your fire
Your mind
Your body
Your aura
Your light

Your everything.
You **are** everything.

You are something to love.

Accepting Love

Accepting love may come easier once you've become
accustomed to expressing love towards yourself.

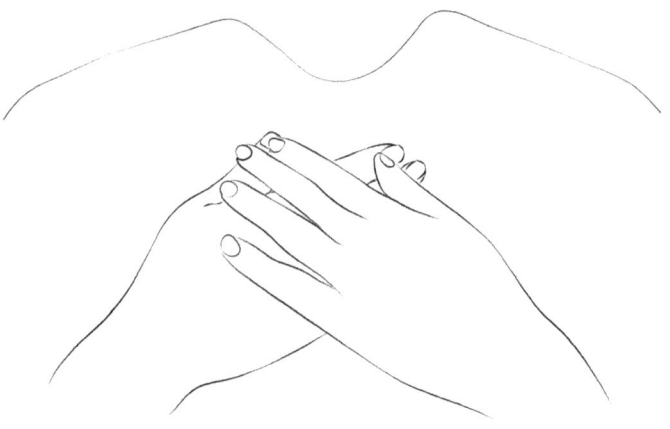

When it comes to love - whether from someone new or
a mended relationship - accepting it can be hard.

It's okay to let people in.

It's okay to give people a chance
to get to know you,
to bring more happiness
into your life.

Remember your boundaries and **trust** yourself
and your intuition.

If someone's offering love
that you would like to experience,
allow **yourself** a chance
to *feel* it.

You don't hide from what you want anymore.

You are *allowed* to feel.

Let it Go

At the risk of coming off harsh,
I think you can handle this:

> Let it go.

> Let *everything* go.

At this point in your journey, it is time to move on from the negativity of your past. The things that once tore you down are no longer relevant when it comes to your wellbeing.

They can cross your mind or come up in conversation but they are

> far gone

> behind you now.

You've come so far - they can't catch up to you now.

You are unstoppable now.

You are free.

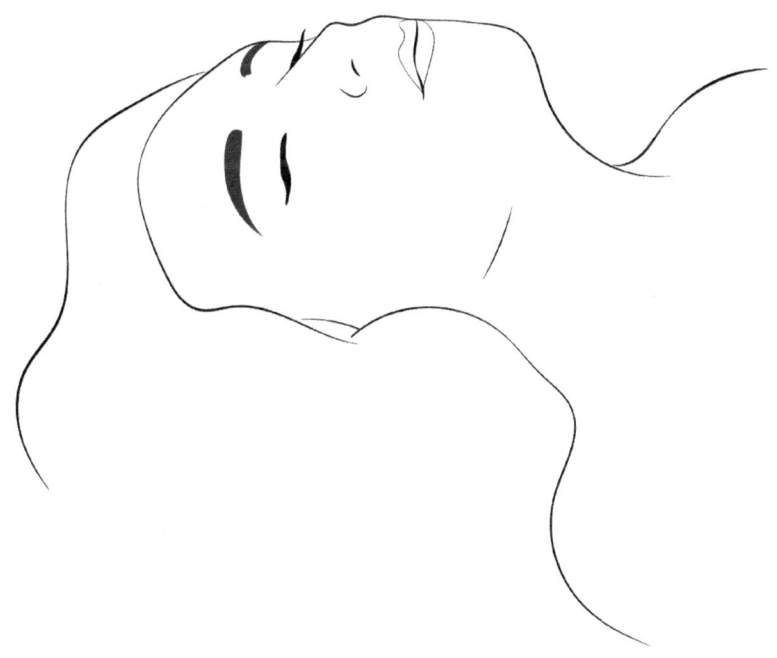

A Home Within Yourself

Home.

This safe place that you have made inside of you is

>*sweet,*
>>*gentle,*
>>>*strong,*
>>>>*loving,*
>>>>>*and warm.*

>It's a perfect place to find comfort.

This is where you feel special and solid but free to be yourself.

Here, you can continue to build, and luckily you are its core and foundation.

>>>If you get a little lost along the way, you can return to this book to help guide you back; but you,

>*you are home.*

If you get a little lost

Remember

You are strong.
It took a lot of strength to relive the memories of your past. It wasn't easy to look at these things from a different perspective. Your strength to face past traumas and move forward is beyond admirable.

You are capable.
No matter what has been said or taught to you, you may have come to realize that you were always capable of so much more...

You are capable of surviving hardships. You are capable of forgiving, accepting, and loving others. More importantly, you are capable of doing these things for yourself. You can surprise yourself everyday with the things you continue to accomplish.

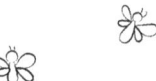

You are special.
You are one of a kind. There is no one else in this world that is like you.

You are amazing.
There is something that is just so beautiful about the way you've been able to make it this far. It's been a long journey and being here now is something to be proud of.

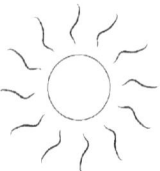

You are more than.
You must always remember that you are *more than* your past. You are more than what people expect of you. You are more than your job, your surroundings, and your social life. You are a person - with actual feelings - that is entitled to some peace, understanding, and respect.

You are always evolving.
This book may have helped you to reconnect with a great part of yourself. As life goes on, we keep growing. There's more to you than what you see now.

You are human.
It is normal to feel a little down sometimes. Just try to avoid **constantly** feeling this way. Attempt to make room for moments of excitement or joy.

You are free.
You no longer hold on to the weight created by a lifetime of trauma. Even though it is a part of you - it doesn't define you. The choices and outcomes of the past don't control your mental wellbeing now.

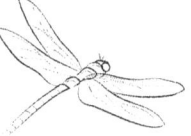

You are worthy.
You deserve more out of life. You are worthy of great things and a better future.

You are light and its vessel.
There are good things inside of you. Love, acceptance, and **willpower** are only a few of your highlights.

You are home.
Anything good that comes your way is a plus.

A Message

Message from the Writer

*I created this journey
while entering it.*

After years,
of bottling in so much
and handling things
in a way
that would keep my anger alive

- to fuel me up and motivate me -

I decided to try
a different way,
with healing
and feeling
whole
to be my new
guide.

*My desire to help others
lays here in these pages.*

This was written
for you.

Glossary

Glossary

Aura
Referring to your energy and vibe. (page 59)

Baggage
Referring to unnecessary weight that has been carried for a long time. (page 22)

Bareness
Referring to feeling vulnerable and without protection. (page 4)

Bottling things up
Referring to holding on to negative thoughts and feelings. (page 24)

Boundaries
Referring to limitations set for yourself and others, to keep you feeling safe and whole. (page 29)

Burden
Referring to the heaviness and weight felt because of a situation or problem. (page 19)

Comfort zone
A place that feels safe and comfortable to you.
In this page, I was referring to a natural and comfortable state of being that you had as a child. (page 3)

Darkness
Referring to dark or negative thoughts. (page 31)

Firecracker
Someone with a strong personality.
This could mean someone that is naturally very hyper, outspoken, or loud. (page 3)

Flame and sparks
Referring to the bright light (or good qualities) you hold inside of you. (page 30)

Home
Referring to you as your place of comfort and stability. (page 64)

Humble
To refrain from feeling or acting superior to others. (page 8)

Inner child
The part of you connected to your younger, more innocent self. This can include your youngest memories - the memories that you still feel connected to in a way that make you feel like you are still that young child. (page 3)

Less than
Referring to someone feeling like less of a person because of someone else's words or actions. (page 42)

Light
Referring to you being able to shine, even in darkness. (page 28)

Mantra
Referring to something that can get you through the day - that can be repeated over and over again. (page 28)

More than
Referring to you as more than all of the things that have been weighing you down. (page 28)

Self
Referring to a version of yourself. (page 4)

Self Sabotage
Referring to self destructive behavior.
More specifically, referring to actions that you take that end up setting you back or causing you harm. These actions may or may not be done consciously. (page 55)

Sit right
Referring to something that does not feel right to you. (page 29)

Them
Referring to him or her.
Words like them, themselves, their, and they are used to refer to the reader. (page 4)

Toxicity
Referring to the result of someone constantly being harsh or toxic towards themselves, resulting in a harmful state of being. (page 24)

Triggers
Referring to a situation, setting, or person that reminds you of past trauma. (page 50)

Unwind
To relax. (page 38)

Vibe
Referring to the energy that you share with others by just being yourself. (page 31)

Vulnerability
Referring to feeling unprotected and unguarded. (page 4)

Willpower
Referring to your ability to continue to move forward. (page 71)

I've left some pages blank for you.

The next pages can be used for
notes, scribbles, thoughts.

*If you wish to pass the book on to a loved one,
the next pages can be used to write them a little note.*

www.ingramcontent.com/pod-product-compliance
Lightning Source LLC
Chambersburg PA
CBHW070623050426
42450CB00011B/3115